DOCTOR
TO
DOCTOR

*Clear Answers
to Your Patients'
Questions about
Noni Juice*

Doctor to Doctor
Direct Source Publishing
15 E. 400 S.
Orem, Ut 84058

TAHITIAN NONI® Juice is a registered trademark of Morinda, Inc.

For questions or comments concerning noni use directed to the author, please send correspondence to the above address.

No information contained here is meant to replace the advice of a doctor or healthcare practitioner. The data and opinions appearing in this book are for informational purposes only. Dr. Neil Solomon does not offer medical advice, and he encourages readers to seek advice from qualified health professionals.

ISBN   1-887938-91-5

DEDICATION

I dedicate this book to the love of my life—my dear wife, Frema, who makes me very happy. To our three special sons and their wives: Ted and Esther, Scott and Florita, and Cliff and Bernadette. And to our precious grandchildren: Scott, Jacob, Bayard, Tessa Grace, and Isabella Rose.

TABLE OF CONTENTS

ACKNOWLEDGMENTS

So many good and trusted colleagues and friends have helped contribute to this work. There are too many to recognize in this limited space. However, I will touch on a few names.

I want to thank Lois Brown for her expertise in research and editing. In addition, I want to thank the following health professionals for sharing their knowledge of noni with me. They include: Bert Acosta, MD; Alan Bailey; Bryant Bloss, M.D.; Dr. Cliff Blumberg; Richard T. Dicks; William Doell, D.O.; Robert Fischer, MD; Dr. Bret Frame; Joel Fuhrman, MD; Dr. Eiichi Furusawa; Dr. Charles Garneir; Scott Gerson, M.D.; Steven Hall, M.D.; Mona Harrison, M.D.; Dr. Delbert Hatton; Dr. Ralph Heinicke; Dr. Tomo Hiramatsu; Dr. Anne Hirazumi Kim; Dr. Samuel Kolodney; Haruhiko Kugo, M.D.; Peter Lodewich, M.D.; Dr. Jim Marcoux; Dr. W.T. Meier; John Mike, M.D.; Susan Mike, M.D.; Dr. Joel Murphy; Maria Odegbaro, MD; Richard Passwater, Ph.D.; Orlando Pile, M.D.; Dr. Nathan Rabb; Dr. Nelson T. Rivers; Larry Scott; Keith Sehnert, M.D.; Dr. Kenneth Stejskal; Dr. Rick T. Smith; Dr. Roger Soard; Dr. T. L. Bryant Taylor; Gary Tran, D.V.M.; Dr. Thomas Velleff; and Mian-Ying Wang, M.D.

I owe many thanks to Jarakae Jensen, Dr. Chen Shu, Jonathan Fritz, and others for sharing their expert scientific and research knowledge about noni; and to Doug McAllister for his professional guidance. Thanks to the many individuals such as John Dilley, Ernie Miller, and Grace Aguliera who shared their personal experiences with noni. Thanks to Jan and Peter Skelly for their continued help in collecting testimonials. Thanks to Colby Allen and McKinley Oswald for their continued confidence. And thanks to Frema Solomon, M.M.H., my agent and editor who also helped in so many ways.

ABOUT THE AUTHOR

Dr. Neil Solomon treated patients for over thirty years before retiring from practicing medicine. He received his AB, MD, and MS degrees from Case-Western Reserve University School of Medicine, Cleveland, Ohio; and clinical training in Medicine on the Osier Medical Service of the Johns Hopkins Hospital, Baltimore, Maryland. He received his Ph.D. from the University of Maryland after completing his Internal Medicine residency training at the Johns Hopkins Hospital.

He has held academic positions such as Assistant Professor at The Johns Hopkins Medical School, and Associate Professor of Physiology and Assistant Professor of Medicine at the University of Maryland School of Medicine.

He did research at the National Institute of Health, National Heart Institute, Department of Gerontology. He was Assistant Senior-Surgeon and Lt. Commander, United States Public Health Service (USPHS). In addition, he served as an Advisor to President Richard Nixon on the Transition Committee, Health Affairs, in Washington, DC. He was also an Advisor to the Secretary of Health, Education and Welfare, in Washington, DC.

Since 1999, Dr. Solomon has been Director of the International Council of Caring Community's (ICCC's) Health Council Advisory Board, a Non Government Organization (NGO) of the United Nations.

Dr. Solomon is a *New York Times* Best Selling Author and for eighteen years was a Syndicated Medical columnist for the *Los Angeles Times* Syndicate.

His many Honors and Awards include: Alpha Omega Alpha, Aaron Brown Scholastic Prize [National Phi Delta Epsilon], Schwentker Award for Outstanding research from the Johns Hopkins Hospital, Maryland Public Health Association Award, Fellow of the Society of Rusk Physicians, Professors and friends in conjunction with RUSK WITHOUT WALLS.

Dr. Solomon's published works include over one hundred articles and books. A portion of these works are listed under Appendix A found at the back of this book.

INTRODUCTION

Dear Colleague,

Like many of you, I had excellent training in traditional medicine, but I had little formal medical school training in alternative medicine. From my days as an undergraduate student at Ohio State University, to my medical school days at Case-Western Reserve University, and to my internal medicine internship and residency training days on the Osler Medical service of the Johns Hopkins Hospital, I studied hard, and kept an open mind, in order to later help my patients. During my more than thirty years of private practice, and as a global health and nutrition consultant, I have continued to strive to help others understand their health problems.

In my recent years, I have come to realize there is more to health and well-being than traditional medicine can offer alone. I believe there is a gap between conventional and alternative medicine. This gap needs to close. Both fields of medicine are legitimate and substantial. Neither field is perfect, but both are striving for the same goal—to deliver a better life to all who seek it.

Over the last six years, I have investigated the healing properties of a tropical plant, Morinda citrifolia, which is largely unknown to most Americans. I believe the fruit from this plant can make a valuable contribution to how physicians can achieve and maintain an improved state of health for their patients. This fruit goes by the interesting, everyday name of noni.

DOCTOR TO DOCTOR

Though I was formally trained as a medical doctor in conventional medicine, I eventually valued so-called "holistic" or "alternative" avenues of medicine. I have always believed that good health began with good nutrition and regular exercise, constructed upon a strong spiritual base.

Even with my openness to alternative medicine, my initial introduction to noni was probably similar to that of many of you. I was skeptical. But it did trigger my interest. I decided to investigate. I began studying medical literature to see what science knew about noni—where it came from, where it grew, how it had been used historically, what studies had been completed regarding its healing value, and what did other medical professionals think about it.

I started contacting everyone I knew who knew anything about noni. Among those I contacted were doctors, nurses, scientists, nutritionists, and a host of other health professionals. The feedback I collected from them spurred me to collect as much information as I could about noni. What I found has transformed my experience with noni into something impressive and rewarding.

Since we have similar medical backgrounds, I assume that you too have asked yourself similar questions. In this book, I plan to answer these questions and other questions you may have concerning the use of noni and exactly what it is.

My hope is that my years of studying and learning about this natural food supplement will save you much of the time and effort I have exerted, but leave you with the same respect and awe for this fruit that I now have.

Best,

Neil Solomon, MD, Ph.D.

SECTION I

What is TAHITIAN NONI® Juice?

"TAHITIAN NONI® Juice is a must for anyone concerned about their well-being. I have taken the juice three to four times a day for nearly a year now. I've noticed so many benefits, and I feel great. Being concerned about my health, and given one supplement of any kind to keep, I'd keep TAHITIAN NONI® Juice, even if it meant moving to Tahiti!"— Dr. Roger Soard, Winchester Bay, Oregon

TAHITIAN NONI® Juice is the brand name for a noni juice that is grown, picked, and bottled in Tahiti by a Utah-based company called Morinda, Inc. In this book, I refer exclusively to TAHITIAN NONI® Juice because Morinda has about 95 percent of the world market of noni juice, and the bulk of the current research was done on TAHITIAN NONI® Juice. Morinda also implements strong quality control measures, and therefore, I feel confident that in referring to this product I will not be leading anyone to an inferior product that may or may not have contaminants.

TAHITIAN NONI® Juice was brought for commercial use into the United States during the mid-nineties by some of the founders of Morinda, Inc. Before that time, few Americans had ever heard of the fruit. However, in Tahiti and in other areas of Polynesia, people had been using noni to promote health and wellness for over 2,000 years.

Noni, or *Morinda citrifolia*, comes from the family Rubiaceae. The noni fruit grows on a small shrub-like tree. The ripened fruit has a green, almost translucent, bumpy skin, and gives off a pungent odor. Noni has been found growing in many islands of the South Pacific (including Hawaii and Tahiti), Malaysia, Indonesia, Taiwan, the Philippines, Vietnam, India, Africa, Guam, and the West Indies. (See Figure 1.)[1]

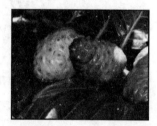

**Figure 1.
Picture of noni fruit**

Historically, the natives used the entire plant for a wide range of therapeutic benefits. Early studies of the plant document that its traditional uses ranged from using the root as a fever-reducing agent, to helping control diabetes, as well as applying the leaves on wounds and ulcers. The fruit had many other ancient medicinal uses that were quite varied. Table 1 lists many of the ailments for which ancient Polynesian healers (called *Kahunas*) used noni.

Table 1. Uses of Noni by Polynesian Healers [2]

Diarrhea	Sore Throat, (Pharyngitis)
Intestinal Worms	Thrush
Cough	Toothache
Chest Cold	Skin Abscess
Pleurisy	Centipede Bite
Tuberculosis	Elephantiasis
Eye Infection (Sty)	Dark Spots
Conjunctivitis	Wounds
Fever	Jaundice
Vomiting	Rheumatism
Inflamed, Sore Gums	Female Problems

Through extensive library research, Dr. Anne Hirazumi Kim catalogued and published the more than 150 nutraceuticals found in noni. These nutraceuticals are listed in Table 2. [3]

Table 2. Nutraceuticals identified in noni

1-butanol
1-hexenol
1-methoxy-2-formyl-3-hydroxy anthraquinone
2,5-undecadien-1-ol
2-heptan one
2-methyl-2-butanoyl decanoate
2-methyl-2-butanoyl hexanoate
2-methyl-3,5,6-trihydroxyanthraquinone-6-§-primeveroside
2-methyl-3,5,6-trihydroxyanthraquinones
2-methyl butanoic acid
2-methylpropanoic acid
24-methylcycloartanol
24-methylene cholesterol
24-methylenecycloartanyl linoleate
3-hydroxyl-2-Butazone
3-hydroxymorindone
3-hydroxymorindone-6-§-primeveroside
3-methyl-2-buten-1-ol
3-methyl-3-buten-1-ol
3-methylthiopropanoic acid
5,6-dihydroxylucidin
5,6-dihydroxylucidin-3-§-primeveroside
5,7-acacetin7-O-§-D-(+)-gluco pyranoside
5,7-dimethyl apigenin-4Õ-O-§-D-D(+)-(galactopyranoside
6,8-dimethoxy-3-methyl anthraquinone-1,-O-§-rhamnosyl gluco pyranoside
6-dodecanoic-y-lactone
7-hydroxy-8-methoxy-2-methyl anthraquinone
8,11,14-eicosatrienoic acid
ascorbic acid
anthocyanadins
acetic acid
alizarin
alkaloids
anthragallol1,2-dimethyl ether
anthraquinones
anthragallol2,3-dimethyl ether
asperuloside
benzoic acid
benzyl alcohol
butanoic acid
calcium
campesteryl glycoside
campesteryl linoleic

glycoside
campesteryl palmitate
campesteryl palmityl
glycoside
campesterol
capric acid
caprylic acid
carbonate
carotene
cycloartenol
cycloartenol linoleate
cycloartenol palmitate
damnacanthal
decanoic acid
elaidic acid
ethyl decanoate
ethyl hexanoate
ethyl octanoate
ethyl palmitate
eugenol
ferric iron
gampesteryl linoleate
glucose
glycosides
heptanoic acid
hexadecane
hexa-amide
hexanedioic acid
hexanoic acid
hexose

hexyl hexanoate
iron
isobutyric acid
iso caproic acid
iso fucosterol
isofucosteryl linoleate
isovaleric acid
lauric acid
limonene
linoleic acid
lucidum
lucidum-3- §-primeveroside
magnesium
methyl3-methylthio-
propanoate
methyl decanoate
methyl elaidate
methyl hexanoate
methyl octanoate
methyl oleate
methyl palmitate
morenone-1
morenone-2
morindadiol
morindanigrine
morindin
morindone
morindone-6-§-primeveroside
mucilaginous matter
myristic acid

n-butyric acid
n-valeric acid
nonanoic acid
nordamnacanthal
octadecanoic acid
octanoic acid
oleic acid
palmitic acid
paraffin
pectins
pentose
phenolic body
phosphate
physcion
physcion-8-O [{L-
proanthocyanadins
arabinopyranosyl}(1-3){§-D-
g-D- galactopyranosyl (1-6)
{§-D- galactopyranoside}]
potassium
protein
proxeronine
proxeroninease
resins
rhamnose
ricinoleic acid
rubiadin
rubiadin-1-methyl ether
rutin*
scopoletin
sitosterol

sitosteryl glycoside
sitosteryl linoleate
sitosteryl linoleyl glycoside
sitosteryl palmitate
sitosteryl palmityl glycoside
sodium
sorandjidiol
§-sitosterol
stearic acid
sterols
stigmasterol
stigmasteryl glycoside
stigmasteryl linoleate
stigmasteryl linoleyl
glycoside
stigmasteryl palmitate
stigmasteryl palmityl
glycoside
terpenoids
trioxymethylanthraquinone
undecenoic acid
ursolic acid
xeronine

Taken with permission from Dr. Hirazumi Kim's work and modified by author.

*Recent findings by Dr. Wang and colleagues at Rutgers have identified for the first time in noni a substance called rutin.

Included in these 150 nutraceuticals are some of the most powerful antioxidants known such as proanthocyanadins, anthocyanadins, vitamin C, and many others.

Quality control is of the utmost importance for any natural supplement, and that holds true for TAHITIAN NONI® Juice. Strict quality control measures give added assurance that TAHITIAN NONI® Juice is safe for children, adults, pregnant and lactating women, and the elderly. TAHITIAN NONI® Juice is tested for over 300 toxins and is thermally pasteurized to maintain its purity.

Table 3 is the nutritional content specifically for TAHITIAN NONI® Juice. The juice contains about 90 percent reconstituted *Morinda citrifolia* fruit juice made from pure juice puree from French Polynesia. The remaining 10 percent is pure, natural grape and blueberry juice for added flavor.. This nutritional information may be important to review with your patients who have diabetes or who suffer from end-stage renal failure where high levels of potassium may cause cardiac arrest. TAHITIAN NONI® Juice contains 28.52 milligrams of potassium per ounce—less than half of the potassium level found in an ounce of orange juice or tomato juice. It is also less than the amount of potassium found in one ounce of apple, grape, or pineapple juice.

Table 3. TAHITIAN NONI® Juice Nutritional Information

Vitamin and Mineral Content for One Serving (1 fluid ounce):		
Vitamins	**Amount**	**% RDA‡**
Biotin	1.47 mcg	0.49%
Folic Acid	7.35 mcg	1.84%
Niacin	0.147 mg	0.735%
Pantothenic Acid	0.147 mcg	1.47%
Vitamin A	5.88 IU	0.117%
Vitamin B1	0.0029 mg	0.196%
Vitamin B12	0.097 mcg	1.62%
Vitamin B2	0.0029 mg	0.17%
Vitamin B6	0.038 mg	1.91%
Vitamin C	6.029 mg	10%
Vitamin E	0.235 IU	0.78%
Minerals	**Amount**	**% RDA‡**
Calcium	6.76 mg	0.67%
Chromium	0.147 mg	no established value
Copper	0.006 mg	0.294%
Iron	0.1088 mg	0.6%
Magnesium	3.088 mg	0.772%
Molybdenum	0.294 mg	no established value
Phosphorus	2.058 mg	0.205%
Potassium	28.52 mg	no established value
Sodium	12.35 mg	no established value
Zinc	0.047 mg	0.313%

Carbohydrate Content for One Serving (1 fluid ounce):		
Carbohydrate	**Amount**	**% RDA‡**
Fructose	1.2 grams	no established value
Glucose	1.1 grams	no established value
Fiber	0.7 grams	no established value

†There is very little fat or protein in TAHITIAN NONI® Juice.
‡Less than 2% of the RDA is not a significant source for this vitamin or mineral.
Used with permission from Morinda, Inc.

In order to ensure that the product they manufacture is contaminant free and of high quality, Morinda has developed what they term a product "footprint." In essence, the footprint is a graphic representation of its proprietary noni juice formula. The peaks of the footprint represent key chemical components that are present.

Now that you know what noni was used for millennia ago, and its ingredients and nutritional value, let's move on to learn about what scientists and researchers have been learning about the juice in recent years.

SECTION II

Scientific Review of the Literature about Morinda Citrifolia

"Thousands of lives are being touched in a positive way, every day by TAHITIAN NONI® Juice. This is the greatest natural product I have ever come across, and perhaps the biggest health breakthrough in decades. I believe it will continue to help many, many people now and in the future."—Dr. Nelson P. Rivers, Pharmacist; Evansville, Indiana

Ever since we have had laboratories and test tubes, scientists have been looking at natural substances to either prove or disprove ancient claims. While no one had brought noni into the United States to sell as a commercial product until the 1990s, some scientists and researchers had heard of noni and were curious about the plant's medicinal claims. One researcher, Dr. Ralph Heinicke, has been analyzing and studying some of the components found in noni and pineapple juice since the 1960s. He has dedicated his life to study noni juice. We will discuss the findings of Dr. Heinicke's work in a later section.

Others started studying noni as early as the mid 20th century. In 1950, O.A. Bushnell published an article in the journal of *Pacific Science* that investigated the antibacterial properties of some lesser-known Hawaiian plants—one such plant was noni.[4] The next decade produced other studies by other scientists. I will discuss two studies of particular interest. The first study, done by Tabrah and Eveleth, was published in the *Hawaiian Medical Journal* and showed the effectiveness of ancient Hawaiian medicine, under which noni fell. Tribunal medical doctors had used the plant for quite some time.[5] The second study, done in 1967, focused singularly on *Morinda citrifolia* and was conducted by K.K. Agarwal. In the study, Agarwal analyzed an extract of Morinda citrifolia (noni), and studied its possible pharmacological uses. The results were preliminary, but positive.[6]

Moving into the 70s and 80s, noni continued to provoke the curiosity of more researchers. A researcher named Oscar Levand studied the plant in graduate school and wrote a dissertation about it. Later, in 1979, he published with a colleague an article in *Planta Medica*. In the article, the researchers pinpoint important chemical constituents in noni that are perhaps what makes the Polynesian wonder such a useful medicinal plant.[7] Two other researchers during the 80s, Abbott and Shimazu, published an article in the *Journal of Ethnopharmacology* about the origins and historical justification for using some unique Polynesian plants in medicine.[8]

These articles and others have helped create an important base for the explosion of research that has come in the 1990s about noni. Many of these earlier articles were not specific in nature as to the diseases that the constituents in noni helped correct. However, in the 1990s, there have been very specific studies done with some positive results. These studies have dealt with TAHITIAN NONI® Juice in connection with hypertension, arthritis, inflammation, pain, cancer, tuberculosis, regeneration of new cells and the repair of sick ones. Let's systematically cover what researchers have learned in these areas.

Hypertension

It is not unreasonable to estimate that as many as half of your patients suffer in some way from cardio-vascular disease. Some of your patients may have had heart attacks; many have high cholesterol and other hyperlipidemias. Undoubtedly you write prescriptions daily for some sort of diuretic or other antihypertensive medications. Heart disease has become a near epidemic, particularly in the United States.

As you are well aware, hypertension has multifactor etiology. It is clear that diet, exercise, and genetics play a role in the human body's circulatory function. However, many people are controlling their diet and exercising regularly, yet they still suffer from high blood pressure.

Modern science is still looking for more answers to why high blood pressure occurs. One such theory centers on a chemical called nitric oxide. In a briefing prepared for the *Royal Society and Association of British Science* writers, it was concluded that:

"Summary research papers continue to flood the scientific journals with insights into the biological activity and potential clinical uses of nitric oxide (NO), a gas that controls a seemingly limitless range of functions in the body. Each revelation adds to nitric oxide's already lengthy résumé in controlling the circulation of the blood, regulating activities of the brain, lungs, liver, kidneys, stomach, and other organs."

The crux of the presentation indicated that the level of nitric oxide is believed to be one controller of blood pressure within the body. Since that time, the 1998 Nobel Prize in Medicine and Physiology was given to three pharmacologists, Drs. Louis J. Ignarro, Ferid Murad, and Robert F. Furchgott, for their work on nitric oxide's role with communication between cells.

Recent studies have shown how specific extracts from *Morinda citrifolia* produce a significant nitric oxide effect in endothelial cells in vitro.[9] It is believed this reaction may be calcium dependent.

Dr. Anne Hirazumi Kim published in vitro data to show the stimulation of the nitric oxide production from noni. The noni effect may be in part the result of the pure air and the calcium-rich soil conditions in which Tahitian noni is grown. TAHITIAN NONI® Juice may enhance the NO effect and provide natural nutrients unmatched in soils of lower quality or less pure air.

In addition to the link between nitric oxide and blood pressure, medical research suggests the possible necessity and importance of nitric oxide in pain relief, diabetes, cancer, stroke, viral and parasitic disease, sunburn, skin disorders, male impotence, and in memory and learning disorders. It may also play a role in many pathological conditions. The varied illnesses that are affected by nitric oxide also seem to be affected (in a positive way) by noni. One doctor, Dr. Maria Odegbaro, M.D., a graduate of the City University of New York Medical School, writes how she has seen noni affect some of the patients in her practice:

While I was training at Waterbury Hospital in Connecticut, my husband, who was an Education Administrator for the New York City Board of Education, was diagnosed with liver cancer. I gathered information on all the clinical trials going on in the Tri-state area on liver cancer, however we ended up at the Cooper University Teaching Hospital in Camden New Jersey with Dr. Order–an authority on liver cancer. Ten weeks later my husband died. It was this tragedy that sparked my interest in alternative medicine.

We now have a clinic in memory of my husband where we help patients to improve their health by monitoring their nutrition in combination with the use of natural products. I have been on several radio and television stations such as WLIB, WHBA, WWRL and Manhattan Cable, during which I appealed to medical schools to start including the natural approach in their training and expand their curriculum to include more courses in nutrition. I am constantly invited to give lectures on alternative medicine at colleges, community centers and churches, such as The Harlem State Health, Holistic Health Watch, and The Natural Way Health for the Community.

In my experience with different natural products, noni tops them all! Patients are faxing me their testimonials everyday. They are reporting results of relief from a variety of conditions such as diabetes, high blood pressure, persistent coughs, asthma, cancer, chronic fatigue syndrome, and arthritis to name a few.

I particularly like the mechanism by which I believe noni works. It stimulates and boosts the body's immune system, therefore enabling the body to produce those substances in the body [such as nitric oxide] that help the body heal itself.[10]

Another key component found in noni that has been connected to lowering blood pressure is scopoletin. In animal studies, scopoletin has been shown to decrease hypertension. In 1993, researchers from the University of Hawaii extracted natural scopoletin from the noni plant. Dr. Isabelle Abbott, a recognized expert in botanical sciences, believes scopoletin is almost certainly involved in the body's response to noni's effect on lowering high blood pressure.[11]

The anecdotal connection between noni and the lowering of high blood pressure is well documented through many personal stories. Take for example John Dilley. John started drinking TAHITIAN NONI® Juice in December of 1998. When he first started drinking noni juice, he hoped it would help with his arthritic shoulders. Within several months the arthritis in his shoulders had disappeared. As a side benefit—and one that many experience while drinking noni juice—he was able to cut his blood pressure medication to one-third of the original dosage within four months of starting noni. He had been on high blood pressure medication for twenty-five years.

Hearing and seeing many similar stories, Scott Gerson, M.D., of the Mt. Sinai School of Medicine in New York, completed a placebo-controlled clinical trial to determine whether noni really could lower high blood pressure in people. For fourteen weeks Dr.

Gerson studied nine hypertensive patients—six males and three females. These patients were selected at random and did not know that they were taking a noni extract.[12]

The patients stayed on the same diet and maintained the same exercise regimens previous to their beginning the trial test. After fourteen weeks of noni treatment, eight of the nine patients showed a significant decrease in blood pressure. On average, their systolic pressure dropped by almost 8 percent, and their diastolic pressure decreased by 4 percent.

While this clinical trial was just that—a clinical trial—it does suggest a possible link between TAHITIAN NONI® Juice and lowering high blood pressure. Nitric oxide and scopoletin are probably not the only factors in decreased blood pressure readings. There are other substances in noni that may also play a part in promoting a healthier cardiovascular system. These two substances in particular deserve our attention and further study.

Arthritis, Inflammation, and Pain

The following personal experience is from Dr. Richard Dicks. Dr. Dicks received his medical degree from Bernadean University and he currently uses noni juice with his patients.

I am involved with natural health care primarily because of my son. He has a bone disease and a special kind of arthritis that confine him to a wheelchair. My son has been in tremendous pain since he was very young. As I've looked for answers to help him, I have also found answers for thousands of people.

Noni juice sparked my interest because of its reputation for massive pain relief. In the natural health care field, we face the challenge of not being able to do much for a patient who has moved into an acute or degenerative stage of pain. When I heard about noni juice from a friend, I decided to do my own detective work on it. For eight months I used it myself and gave it to my son without telling anyone. My son's pain dissipated until it was almost gone! We need to get back to the basics with our bodies.[13]

Aspirin, Ibuprofen, Vioxx, or Celebrex, are well known to you and to your many patients who suffer daily from both osteoarthritis and rheumatoid arthritis. As you know, many non-steroidal anti-inflammatory drugs (N-SAIDs) are used to control the pain and swelling that accompany degenerative joint disease. You are also well aware that many of these medications have other side effects that can be as unpleasant as the arthritis.

Even the new and highly acclaimed COX 2 inhibitors, Vioxx, or Celebrex, have their share of negative side effects such as rashes, facial swelling, unusual bleeding, and stomach pain for some people when used continuously. As you also know, antibiotics are used when treating infectious arthritis. Long-term use of antibiotics is well known to have possible negative effects on the body, and the recent development of antibiotic resistant bacteria. None of these conventional medications are usually bad; in fact, in some cases they have been lifesavers.

However, I found that in my experience there was nothing more frustrating than to prescribe a patient a medication and then have her or him come back in a few months with more problems from the medication than from the original problem. Wouldn't it be great to not have to prescribe something you knew could have negative side effects? Of course, that something would have to address the problem. Recent research indicates that TAHITIAN NONI® Juice has a viable and significant effect on the selective inhibition of the COX 2 enzyme that is known to cause inflammation and pain.

As a brief reminder, the COX 1 enzyme produces prostaglandins associated with maintaining the lining of the digestive tract. The COX 2 enzyme produces prostaglandins associated with inflammation and pain. (Table 4.) When treating arthritis, you want to lower the amount of the COX 2 enzyme in the body and not disturb the levels of COX 1. In so doing you reduce the pain without aggravating the stomach.

Table 4. COX 1 vs. COX 2 Comparison

COX 1 (protective enzyme)	COX 2 (pain-inducing enzyme)
• Found in most tissues • Easily identifiable • Protects stomach lining • Important in regulating normal cell function • Gene found on chromosome 9	• Found in increased number in cancer, inflamed, and sick brain cells • Difficult to identify • Causes pain, swelling, and inflammation • Gene found on chromosome 1

In a study conducted at the Morinda Research Laboratory located in Provo, Utah, researchers Dr. Chen Shu, Jonathan Fritz, Jarakae Jensen, and others investigated the effect TAHITIAN NONI® Juice has on COX enzymes. Researchers compared the inhibition ratio of the COX 1 enzyme to the COX 2 enzyme using different products. They discovered that TAHITIAN NONI® Juice has a very favorable inhibition ratio when compared to both over-the-counter and prescription arthritis medications. Boiled down, TAHITIAN NONI® Juice selectively inhibits the COX 2 enzyme that produces prostaglandins associated with inflammation and pain while allowing the COX 1 enzyme to produce prostaglandins associated with maintaining the lining of the digestive tract. The study was repeated and confirmed by two independent labs—one located in France and the other in Taiwan. The actual inhibition ratio can be seen in Table 5.[14]

Table 5. Comparison of IC_{50} Ratios of Several Drugs and TAHITIAN NONI® Juice

Comparison of ratio of inhibition of COX 2/COX 1 (IC_{50} %)	
Product	IC_{50} % ratio
TAHITIAN NONI® Juice	0.35
Celebrex®	0.34
Indomethacin	40
Aspirin	119

Another reason for noni's pain-fighting qualities may stem from several of its constituents. Noni has been shown to contain scopoletin, which has anti-inflammatory effects. Scopoletin is needed in the body for smooth joint movement. It also produces anti-histamine effects. A laboratory in France conducted a study that showed mice, given a liquid form of *Morinda citrifolia*, increased pain tolerance as reflected by their reaction time to a hot plate. The researchers concluded that noni helped the mice better deal with the pain from the hot plate.[15]

The different compounds in noni that affect pain and inflammation have changed the lives of many doctors and the lives of many of their patients as well. The following is the personal experience of Dr. T. L. Bryant Taylor, a practicing bone specialist in Taylor, Michigan:

I had twisted my left knee getting out of the car, causing excruciating pain for several weeks. I was unable to put any weight on the knee because it was too weak and would collapse. In addition to my knee pain, I had a problem with my wrists. I have been practicing for 17 years, and the strain on my wrists from working with patients had left my wrists unable to flex. My right shoulder blade and rotator cuff were also often painful. As a result, I was unable to rest on my right side. I began taking TNJ on 15 December 2001. After drinking the juice for one week, my knee pain was gone and it was able to bear weight. Along with the knee success, I realized that both of my wrists could flex, and that I was able to rest on my right side without any pain.

Many patients have also had great success using noni juice to help with arthritis associated pain. Many of my medical colleagues have shared stories of patients who have experienced pain relief after starting to drink TAHITIAN NONI® Juice. One such person is Ernie Miller.

Ernie is 72 and has had rheumatoid arthritis for about seven years. As medications stopped working, his doctor would change to a new medication. In January 1999, Ernie began drinking noni juice. He had tried many things and was on weekly gold shots, Sulfasalazine pills, and delayed-release aspirin. After six weeks, a big change in Ernie's condition began to take place. At first, he had more energy. Then the stiffness and pain in his joints began to leave. Today, he is able to move his head, arms, and knees without pain! He receives only one gold shot per month and has nearly stopped taking aspirin.

Cancer

Most of the research conducted in the last ten years with TAHITIAN NONI® Juice has been done on the plant's effect on cancerous and pre-cancerous cells. Much of the current knowledge about cancer and TAHITIAN NONI® Juice is due to two researchers— Dr. Anne Hirazumi Kim, and Mian-Ying Wang, M.D.

The laboratory relationship between noni and cancer started in the early 1990s. It was at this time that researchers in both the United States and Japan started investigating what was in the *Morinda citrifolia* plant that seemed to fight off one of the deadliest diseases known—cancer.

In 1992, Dr. Anne Hirazumi Kim presented data from her first study dealing with noni and cancer at a convention for the American Association for Cancer Research. Her laboratory studies were some of the first to show, using a clear scientific method, that noni appeared to slow and even stop cancer in mice suffering from Lewis Lung carcinoma. Later, she wrote an impressive doctoral dissertation on the subject.[16]

She continued her research throughout the 90s, publishing her latest work on the subject in 1999.[17] This most recent work, representing data from Drs. Hirazumi Kim and Furusawa, suggests that noni may suppress cancerous tumor growth by modulating the host's immune system. The doctors hypothesize that noni boosts the body's immune system. The modulated immune system is then able to more efficiently combat cancerous cell invasion. The study showed that in mice there was improved survival time from cancer when noni was added to a "sub-optimal dose" of standard chemotherapeutic agents such as Adriamycin, Cisplatin, and

Vincristine. The researchers believed this data strengthened noni's position as a supplemental agent in cancer treatment. Other articles and research done by Dr. Hirazumi Kim have been published in the *Proceedings of the Western Pharmacological Society.*[18]

Also in the early 90s, scientists in Japan were doing their own independent research. In 1993, four scientists published an article in *Cancer Letters* that validated *Morinda citrifolia's* possible cancer-fighting abilities. In this study, the scientists injected ras cells (cells that are precursors to many malignant growths) with a substance called damnacanthal found in noni roots. They observed that the injection of noni significantly inhibited the ras cells from reproducing.[19] Other studies on noni's effect on tumor necrosis have been published in other countries as well.[20]

Since these earlier studies, a new noni researcher has entered the scene—Mian-Ying Wang, MD, from the University of Illinois Medical School. Before specifically studying noni's effect on cancer, Wang did considerable work with cytokinetics of cancerous cells and how anticancer drugs affect them. She has also studied chemical and hormonal carcinogenesis, and cancer prevention at the initiation stage of cancer development.

However, for the past few years Wang has been aggressively studying the impact TAHITIAN NONI® Juice has on cancer. Wang recently released an intriguing article that pointed to noni's possible preventative effect on cancer. This study showed that mice who were given a solution of 10 percent TAHITIAN NONI®Juice for a week and then injected with DMBA (a known cancer-causing agent) had significantly lower DNA adduct markers (a test for abnormal mutant cells) than mice who were fed only water and then injected with DMBA. The noni-fed mice had 50 percent fewer DNA markers in the lungs than the water-fed mice. In addition, the noni-fed mice had 60 percent fewer markers in the heart, 70 percent fewer markers in the liver, and 90 percent fewer markers in the kidneys. (Figures 1 and 2.)[21] The noni-fed mice had more protection against the cancer-causing agent than the water-fed mice did.

Figure 1. Density of DNA adduct markers in kidney and heart

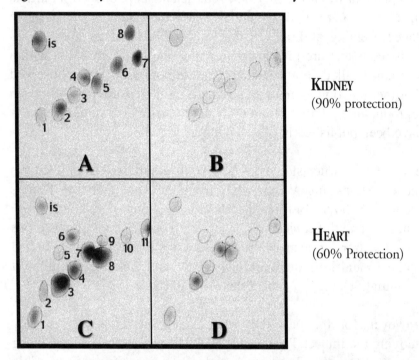

KIDNEY
(90% protection)

HEART
(60% Protection)

Autoradiographic density pattern of DNA adduct markers (single nucleotide) from two-dimensional thin layer chromatography. *These figures show that the density of the markers of the group of rats who took noni as seen on the right side (B and D) is significantly lower than the density of the markers of the group on the left (A and C) who did not drink noni. The lower the density , the more the prevention and protection against cancer.*

Figure 2. Density of DNA adduct markers in liver and lung

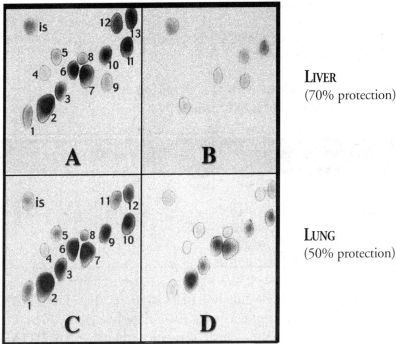

LIVER
(70% protection)

LUNG
(50% protection)

Autoradiographic density pattern of DNA adduct markers (single nucleotide) from two-dimensional thin layer chromatography. *These figures show that the density of the markers of the group of rats who took noni as seen on the right side (B and D) is significantly lower than the density of the markers of the group on the left (A and C) who did not drink noni. The lower the density, the more the prevention and protection against cancer.*

[Figures 1 and 2 and Table 6 were obtained from Dr. Mian-Ying Wang's work and are used here with her permission. Under no circumstances can these figures (or any portions of this book) be photocopied or duplicated in any way without written permission from the publisher.]

Dr. Wang has continued with her research. In 2000, she published the results of her study in the *Annals of the New York Academy of Sciences.*[22] A summation of the latest study completed by Dr. Wang and her associate can be seen in Table 6. Dr. Wang's study addressed the hypothesis of whether TAHITIAN NONI® Juice possesses a cancer preventative effect at the initiation stage of carcinogenesis. Preliminary data suggests that pretreatment for one week with TAHITIAN NONI® Juice in drinking water at a concentration of 10% was able to reduce DMBA-DNA adduct formation (marker for developing cancer) in rats.

Table 6. Pretreatment with rats drinking 10% TAHITIAN NONI® Juice

% Cancer Reduction (Males)		% Cancer Reduction (Females)
Heart	60%	30%
Lungs	50%	41%
Liver	70%	42%
Kidney	90%	80%

From her studies, Dr. Wang not only suggests that TAHITIAN NONI® Juice may prevent cancer at its initiation stage by blocking carcinogen induced DNA adduct formation, but that TAHITIAN NONI® Juice has other cancer-preventing qualities as well. She has shown in vitro and in vivo that TAHITIAN NONI® Juice reduces cancer growth through its scavenging reactive oxidative species (ROS), its quenching lipid peroxides (LPO), and its anti-inflammatory effect.

Even more recently, she has completed a small, one-year pilot study of a double blind human clinical trial on how TAHITIAN NONI® Juice may decrease the DNA damage caused by smoking cigarettes in current smokers. This damage is a pre-cursor to some of the cancers that smokers are known to develop with greater frequency than non-smokers. Results from the pilot study were positive, and now Dr. Wang is continuing this line of research with an even larger number of participants.

Dr. Wang and the others show that the relationship between cancer and noni suggests some very promising results. These investigations into natural supplements are much needed in a world where our fight against cancer remains a major challenge despite the advancements in chemotherapy and radiation treatment. The research studies cited lend credence to the many personal testimonials that I receive from others about noni juice and cancer.

One doctor, who has seen many patients use noni as a supplement adjunct to their cancer treatments, is Dr. Kenneth Stejskal. Dr. Stejskal has been involved with cancer research since 1975. During that time he has associated with over 2,000 doctors worldwide. Since 1972, he has treated over 19,000 patients with different types of illness. Since 1987, when he first began the treatment of terminally ill cancer patients, he has treated around 8,000 terminally ill and he reports losing only 64 patients.[23]

Dr. Stejskal, who has his own clinic, is giving his patients noni juice as one of the nutritional supplements that he feels is important in attacking cancer. He feels noni juice helps to cleanse the body of toxins and supplies the body with the right nutrients. He reports that many of his patients return to him with news that they have completely rid their bodies of breast tumors, brain tumors, and other types of cancerous growths.

Another doctor, family physician Joel Fuhrman, MD, has also seen good results in his practice and with members of his immediate family. He writes:

As a family physician that specializes in nutritional medicine, I have found certain natural products to be helpful for various conditions, especially in combination with aggressive dietary change and optimal nutrition.

I started using noni juice with my patients and never have I seen a product so effective for so many different conditions. To my amazement, noni juice offered relief in the majority of cases for many different conditions. Almost every patient reported pain relief from musculoskeletal symptoms. It worked remarkably well for degenerative joint disease, rheumatoid arthritis, fibromyalgia, and even garden-variety back pain.

My father has chronic lymphocytic leukemia with a steadily worsening anemia and a climbing white blood cell count. After just two weeks on noni, his anemia improved. His white count dropped from 115 to 76. Not only that, but my father had also suffered severe ankle injuries during World War II. After only five days of being on the juice, he could dance pain-free after being in pain for years.

I urge all health professionals to try noni juice on themselves and their patients. I'm convinced it could make a significant difference in most people's health.[24]

Tuberculosis

With the exception of bacteria-resistant strains, tuberculosis is no longer a major health threat in most areas in the United States. But it is still a problem in other, less developed areas of the world. Also, the cases of tuberculosis that do resurface seem to be from drug-resistant strains that don't respond to usual anti-microbial treatment. For these two reasons, researchers have been looking for new ways to combat the disease.

At the 2000 International Chemical Congress of Pacific Basin Societies, researchers from the University of Santo Tomas in Manila, Philippine Islands, presented a study that showed the noni plant had been found to kill the bacterium tuber bacillus, which causes tuberculosis. The American Chemical Society hosted the conference and many scientists from around the world presented their work.

In the Philippine study, researchers found that in laboratory tests a concentration of extracts from the leaves of the noni plant killed 89 percent of the pathogens known to cause tuberculosis. The leading drug, rifampicin, which is a common drug used to treat tuberculosis, killed 97 percent of the pathogens at comparable concentrations.

The active compounds in noni that researchers believe are responsible for the inhibition activity of tuberculosis pathogens are the phytosterols within noni (otherwise known as plant sterols). Noni's phytosterols are structurally different from the other compounds used to treat tuberculosis. Because of this, researchers believe that the compounds within the noni extract are fighting off the pathogens using a different mechanism than the traditional drugs use.[25] (As you know, plant sterols are safe, and shouldn't be confused with "steroids" used in humans.)

These researchers, funded by the Philippine government, the International Foundation for Science, and UNESCO, say that the results are very promising. As a result, they will continue to study the plant, and they encourage pharmaceutical companies to do the same. The team indicated that studies of the different parts of the plant, such as the fruit, are underway.

Cellular Growth and Repair

Reports from fellow medical doctors now pour in about the success some of their patients are experiencing by incorporating noni into their diet. At first, the wide range of these reports turned me off, as they might most medical professionals. The personal stories about the supplement reminded me of a good snake oil that could cure anything. However, the stories kept coming from around the world. Instead of dismissing these reports, I reviewed the research to see if it was possible for one supplement to do so many different things.

One possibility in which noni seems to affect so many bodily systems is through its stimulation of nitric oxide. In an earlier section, we already discussed the varied uses for nitric oxide in the body, and in particular its potential relationship to hypertension.

Another way I believe that noni is able to affect so many systems is through its ability to promote new cellular growth and to repair damaged cells. Everything in our body is made up of cells. An accumulation of damaged cells could result in a damaged organ or system. There are several ways that noni can help rebuild the body's overall cellular growth. To begin, TAHITIAN NONI® Juice is a powerful antioxidant. Much has been written in recent years about cellular damage resulting from *free radicals.*

Free radicals occur when the chains of important biochemicals in the body are broken with a resultant unpaired electron remaining. This occurs because of oxidization in the body. The "radicals" of these broken chains then move around the body as free radicals, causing damage to other cells. When a cell is hit by a free radical, the cell may become more permeable and "leaky," the mitochondria may actually be compromised, or DNA might be damaged. Many scenarios result in a "sick cell." [26]

In order to combat the potential effects of free radicals, the body needs to first prevent oxidization (with an anti-oxidant), and next, it needs something to rebuild the already damaged cells. Studies show that noni can help do both.

In Table 7, the antioxidant activity of TAHITIAN NONI® Juice is compared to the antioxidant activity of several other well-known compounds often used for their ability to prevent free radical damage.

Table 7. Antioxidant Activity (LPO and TNB)

Food Supplements Tested	Prevent free radical damage
TAHITIAN NONI® Juice	*100%
Vitamin C	2.8 X Less
Pycnogenol®	1.4 X Less
GSP	1.1 X Less

LPO = Lipid hydroperoxide quenching activity assay
TNB = Tetrazolium nitroblue, scavenger activity assay
* TAHITIAN NONI® Juice was arbitrarily assigned 100% as the "gold standard," and the potency of other food supplements were tested against it.

In addition to the antioxidant activity in noni, Dr. Ralph Heinicke, Ph.D., has pinpointed constituents in noni that he believes are responsible for the juice's ability to promote cellular growth. These are parts of his postulated xeronine system, which consists of proxeronine, proxeroninease, and xeronine.

In his book, The Xeronine System, Dr. Heinicke outlines how he became what many consider to be one of the world's foremost experts on noni. It began when he was hired on at the Pineapple Research Institute in Hawaii in the early 1950s. His assignment was to find a way to commercially isolate a substance called bromelain. He succeeded in this endeavor. Reports from medical professionals started filtering back to him about the different ways this "impure" form of bromelain helped their patients with skin burns and uterine abnormalities among other things.

Dr. Heinicke concluded there must be some beneficial medicinal properties associated with the bromelain extracts. Hence, he set out to purify the bromelain in order to secure FDA approval. However, every attempt to purify the bromelain resulted in its also losing some of its medicinal therapeutic qualities.

He continued his research for years. He was able to isolate two mysterious crystal compounds from within the "unpurified bromelain." He named these substances proxeronine and xeronine.

He left the Pineapple Research Institute to do similar research for a Japanese company. Years later, Dr. Heinicke once again tried to extract xeronine from pineapple. This time he found that he could not duplicate it. He examined the electrophoretic pattern of the old pineapple fruit grown in Hawaii compared to the new pineapple fruit being grown. He found that the fruits were different. The aggressive treatment of the soil in which pineapple was grown had, over several decades, actually changed the fruit itself.

Dr. Heinicke went looking for other food that would be a natural source of proxeronine and xeronine. He found it at last in noni. Since TAHITIAN NONI® Juice was grown in unhampered soil in Tahiti, the fruit had maintained the important ingredients he believed necessary for cellular enhancement.

In essence, Dr. Heinicke theorizes that the substance in noni called proxeronine, when combined with the enzyme proxeroninease in the body, forms the alkaloid, xeronine. Xeronine, he believes, is a cellular boosting alkaloid that affects nearly every cell and function of the body.[27]

The xeronine theory, which is based on much of Dr. Heinicke's work, postulates that once in the body, proxeronine travels to specific parts of cells, such as the mitochondria, microsomes, Golgi apparatus, reticuloendothelium, electron transport system, DNA, RNA, and etc. Within the cell, these components communicate with each other (intracellular) and with other cells (intercellular). This communication between cells may work according to the theories of several Nobel Prize winning doctors.

In 1998, Nobel Prize laureates in medicine, and doctors of pharmacology, Drs. Robert Fuchgott, Ferid Murad, and Louis Igano demonstrated that nitric oxide allows cells to communicate with each other. Nitric oxide becomes one of their special languages.[28] As already mentioned, noni helps stimulate nitric oxide production.

According to the theory, within these structures, proxeronine combines with other natural biochemicals and building blocks (i.e. hormones, proteins, enzymes, serotonin, vitamins, minerals, and antioxidants). The Golgi apparatus and the reticuloendothelium then assemble all the necessary compounds into a specific "package" and deliver the "package" to the sick parts of the cell, or they may carry the "package" via the blood stream to other sick cells. Rockerfeller University Biologist, Dr. Guenther Blobel, has advanced this "generalized body delivery system". In his work, for which he won the 1999 Nobel Prize, he explained how proteins are shipped to cells using a "postal and zip code" sort of system.[29]

As the receiving sick cell opens the "package" sent by the Golgi apparatus and the reticuloendothelium, the packaged proxeronine combines with another cellular enzyme called proxeroninease. It is postulated that this combination converts into xeronine, which is then used by the body to help rebuild the damaged cells.

The ability of noni to help promote cellular growth is what many doctors attribute to noni's wide range of success. For example, noni has been reported to be successful with some of the hard-to-treat autoimmune disorders. Dr. Delbert Hatton from Washington, D.C., reports success in this area:

I began recommending noni to my patients last fall. Since then I have had nothing but success with it. The most amazing case I know of is a woman with AIDS. Since she has been drinking noni, her T-cell count has gone from 169 to 400 and her symptoms have stabilized. I also have a relative with lung cancer whose tumors have decreased in size since he has been drinking noni.

Several years ago, one of my patients was traumatically injured in an auto accident. He broke several ribs, his shoulder, and his knee. Since then he has had a lot of problems with arthritis, especially in his knee. After he started using noni, the pain in his knee went away immediately and he had a gradual decrease in the pain in his ribs and shoulder. Now he is a happy, pain-free man.

Diabetes is another disease with which many have reported good results after drinking noni juice. One woman, Grace Aguliera, is a Type II diabetic who was required to take insulin shots. Her glucose decreased from 240 to 135 after two weeks of drinking noni juice. Her doctor then prescribed for her an oral medication. Her blood sugar has remained stabilized, and she has been able to stay on oral medication and drink noni juice.

These accounts and others are consistent with the xeronine theory, and to the use of noni as a natural supplement to help strengthen the body and promote overall better health.

SECTION III

What Other Doctors Have to Say about Noni

Once I recognized the wide variety of beneficial effects TAHITIAN NONI® Juice is capable of conferring, I felt compelled to share this product with my patients. I know that TAHITIAN NONI® Juice has helped all of my patients who have tried it, and it can help anyone who is looking to benefit overall. I have directly or indirectly changed the lives of over 2,000 people by introducing them, or someone they know, to TAHITIAN NONI® Juice. My personal results have been nothing short of miraculous. Try it— you'll love it.— Dr. Samuel Kolodney; New Hope, Pennsylvania

As a doctor, it is very hard to know when to try something off the beaten path. The following is a collection of the personal experiences different doctors have had with noni juice. Many were unsure at first whether or not to even give noni a try. Many used the juice on themselves or close family members before daring to introduce it to patients.

Everyone has a different method of feeling comfortable using something not considered a conventional medicine in his or her practice. However, what the overall consensus of these doctors will show is that they are glad they started using noni. And even more important, so are their thousands of patients who have since benefited from its use.

Bert Acosta, MD

Dr. Bert Acosta received his undergraduate degree from the University of California, Davis, and then went on to graduate from Ross University School of Medicine in 1983. He did his residency work at the St. Vincent Hospital in Ohio. He has been in private practice as an internist for fifteen years, and currently he is the medical director of the Noble House Medical Clinic in New Castle, Pennsylvania.

When Dr. Acosta began his private practice in Pennsylvania, he was what some would consider a very "conventional" doctor. Over the course of time, however, he began to notice events that impacted his line of thinking. First, the U.S. government passed a new law cutting back medication reimbursement for senior citizens. As an internist, many of Dr. Acosta's patients were elderly. Dr. Acosta knew that he was writing prescriptions for sickly patients who could never afford to purchase the hundred-dollar medications. He knew these patients would just go home and continue to be sick. Next, Dr. Acosta's parents began to have failing health. Both of them were taking 10 different pills daily; yet, their condition did not improve. He started to earnestly look into what could be done preventatively. Then, about four years ago, he set out on a serious investigative adventure.

This investigation led him on a two-year learning curve of alternative methods. He tried to acquire all the knowledge he could about the field to see if it might possibly be an avenue for some of his patients. During the two years he attended a continuing education seminar on alternative medicine sponsored by Harvard University and the University of San Francisco. It was at these seminars that he finally decided there really was something worthwhile to alternative medicine. One of the natural supplements that were briefly discussed at this convention was the fruit called noni.

A little while later, a colleague introduced Dr. Acosta to the product called TAHITIAN NONI® Juice. First he was skeptical because the claims from those using the product were so far-reaching. However, he decided to use it on his parents. His father suffered from hypertension, diabetes, arthritis, coronary heart disease, and an enlarged prostate. His mother had severe colon problems. Both his mother and father were able to reduce their medication by 50 percent after regularly drinking noni juice. He decided to ask 200 of his patients who were not responding well to the conventional methods he was using with them to try noni juice.

These 200 patients were to use the juice from 30 to 60 days and then return and report how they were doing. Many of the patients reported success and the news spread like wildfire in Dr. Acosta's small town. To date, he is supplementing conventional treatment with noni juice with over 1,200 patients. Dr. Acosta estimates that in his town alone there are now 6,000 people drinking noni juice. He has received some heat from other doctors, but Dr. Acosta says the results he sees in his patients make up for it. On the other hand, some fellow doctors have also started to use the juice supplement.

Dr. Acosta has used the juice in patients with conditions that range from leukemia to diabetes. He says one patient, a young man who came into his office very sick, was diagnosed with leukemia. They tried all of the conventional methods such as bone marrow transplants, blood transfusions, etc., but nothing seemed to help. Dr. Acosta then told the young man about noni. The young man was willing to try it and after six months on the juice, Dr. Acosta reported that the man's leukemia went into remission.

In this particular situation, Dr. Acosta realizes that the man may have gone into remission without noni, even though before taking noni there was no indication of any type of recovery. And while personal experiences like this should not be assumed to be scientific proof, Dr. Acosta has seen many similar scenarios in his practice since he started using noni.

For example, others in Dr. Acosta's practice have used noni juice to help control their diabetes. Dr. Acosta estimates that after drinking TAHITIAN NONI® Juice, over 70 percent of the diabetics in his practice have been able to decrease the amount of diabetic medication they take. In addition, about 100 of his patients with hypertension have also been able to decrease their medication after supplementing their diets with noni. Fifty of his patients have been helped to lose, on average, 10 pounds. Dr. Acosta himself says he has lost 22 pounds without changing his lifestyle except for drinking TAHITIAN NONI® Juice.

Dr. Acosta says he is very comfortable recommending TAHITIAN NONI® Juice as a nutritional supplement. The results have shown that the supplement has had positive effects in approximately 68 percent of all the patients that have used it.

Bryant Bloss, MD

Dr. Bryant Bloss is an orthopedic surgeon who has been in private practice in Indiana since 1963. He received his medical degree from the University of Louisville Medical School. He has been on many professional boards during the last four decades. He has served on the Board of Directors of the Southern Baptist Hospital for seventeen years and was President for four years. He has also served on the Board of Counselors to the American Academy of Orthopedic Surgeons, and was a member of the Executive Committee and editorial committee of the Clinical Orthopaedic Society.

When Dr. Bloss began his private medical practice in 1963, he considered himself a strictly conventional doctor. He had always been interested in rheumatoid arthritis, since his brother had suffered many years from the debilitating disease. In medical school, Dr. Bloss did numerous papers on the subject and particularly studied and wrote about artificial joint replacement.

After being in the medical field for several years, he was asked to be the director of the musculoskeletal clinic that housed nine or ten doctors and physical therapists within the clinic, some of whom were chiropractors. Typically, orthopedic doctors and chiropractors do not work in conjunction with each other. However, in this setting, Dr. Bloss was introduced to "alternative methods." He learned from the other doctors, and they learned from him. Dr.

Bloss recalls the experience as a time during which many eyes were opened.

An optician's office was located next to Dr. Bloss' clinic. This optician introduced Dr. Bloss to a juice supplement called TAHITIAN NONI® Juice. Interested in its arthritic connection, Dr. Bloss first tried the juice on himself. Then he tried it on his family. Other doctors started asking him about it, and some medical professionals under his care started drinking the juice. Currently, 700 of his patients are now drinking TAHITIAN NONI® Juice.

Dr. Bloss has found the juice to be most effective in three specific areas: rheumatoid arthritis, diabetes, and illness caused by smoking. He has seen clients have great success with the juice particularly in these three areas.

One of Dr. Bloss' patients suffered from Ankylosing Spondylitis of the back. The patient could hardly even ride in a car or get out of the house. The patient was taking 3200 milligrams of ibuprofen, 12 Darvocet, and 9 Soma a day. Dr. Bloss added TAHITIAN NONI® Juice to the patient's diet and remarkably within two to three weeks the patient was off the other medication.

Another patient had Sporotrichosis in the knees, wrists, and ankles. Sporotrichosis is an extremely rare fungus infection of joints or bones. This patient also smoked three packs of cigarettes a day and had a blood sugar level of over 600 mgm %. After being on a regimen of TAHITIAN NONI® Juice and other measures, the patient's blood sugar dropped. He quit smoking, and he has not had a recurrence of Sporotrichosis in two and a half years.

Another man had avascular necrosis of the hip, which can be a precursor to arthritis. The ball in his hip joint was dissolving and he would soon have to have a hip replacement. He also had a ruptured disk in his back and was on Celebrex". In addition, the man had high blood pressure and elevated blood cholesterol, and he was taking Lipitor" and blood pressure meds. Dr. Bloss suggested TAHITIAN NONI® Juice. After taking the juice regularly, the man was able to stop taking the Lipitor", blood pressure meds, and Celebrex". The real success is that he now has less pain. His blood pressure is the lowest that he can remember.

On a personal note, Dr. Bloss says his own arthritis improved on TAHITIAN NONI® Juice. As a great side benefit, he has not had a migraine headache in over five years since drinking TAHITIAN NONI® Juice, and had fewer URI's. He anxiously awaits the results of the current Medical University research being done on TAHITIAN NONI® Juice.

Steven Hall, MD

Like many other doctors who have incorporated noni into their medical practice, Dr. Steven Hall's first experience with noni was a personal one. Dr. Hall, a graduate of University of Utah College of Medicine, herniated a disk in a trampoline accident in 1985. In order to control the pain, Dr. Hall tried anything and everything including chiropractic, physical therapy, acupuncture, supplements, yoga, etc. He was able to get some relief from these methods, but the relief was sporadic and unpredictable. In 1995, ten years after the original trampoline accident, Dr. Hall's back went out again. X-rays of the area showed he had developed degenerative problems. He began experiencing numbness in his left foot and muscle spasms.

Then, in the fall of 1996, Dr. Hall's wife bought two bottles of TAHITIAN NONI® Juice from a friend. She asked her husband to try drinking just one ounce of juice twice a day. Dr. Hall agreed, seeing nothing to lose. He almost immediately noticed a change for the better in his energy level. Three weeks after starting the juice, Dr. Hall remembers calling his wife at home and telling her that he hadn't thought of his back all day. Things continued to look up for him. His back spasms decreased and then went away altogether. He could tell there was still arthritis in his back, but gentle stretching and physical therapy started to reliably help instead of sometimes helping, and sometimes hurting.

Three months after being on TAHITIAN NONI® Juice, the sense of feeling returned to Dr. Hall's left foot. At first his foot felt like it was waking up from sitting crossed-legged on the floor too long. Then, a completely normal feeling returned. Seeing her husband's success, Dr. Hall's wife also started drinking noni juice and was able to better control migraines from which she had suffered for years.

The clincher for Dr. Hall came when he began giving his toddler son TAHITIAN NONI® Juice. His son would have grand mal seizures whenever he fell and hit his head. Dr. Hall had his son evaluated by a pediatric neurologist. The evaluation came back as normal, but anti-seizure medication was prescribed as a precaution. Dr. Hall knew the negative effects of the anti-seizure medication. Before starting his son on the medication, he decided to start researching noni in earnest.

His search lead him to medical literature, ethnobotany literature, and some one-on-one talks with Dr. Ralph Heinicke. After doing the research, Dr. Hall concluded that there was nothing in noni that would hurt his son, and the cellular enhancing qualities of noni just might help with the seizure problem. Dr. Hall's son started with just one ounce a day. He loved the juice. He would ask for it by name. He has had no more seizures, and has been a very healthy child, avoiding many of the ear infections experienced by his older siblings.

While doing his extensive research, Dr. Hall realized he had a medical practice full of people who could benefit form noni. He considered the option of telling his patients about noni for a while. He did some real soul-searching and at last decided he felt comfortable sharing what he had found with his patients. His medical practice has a lot of patients who have been to Western specialists as well as alternative practitioners and who still have problems. Dr. Hall uses a combination approach that really focuses on treating the whole person and not just symptoms.

Since that time, Dr. Hall has seen benefits using the juice with over 600 of his patients. He has been practicing medicine for seventeen years. He has published a book, *Noni Through Your Body*, which documents what he has learned about noni.[30]

Mona Harrison, MD

Dr. Mona Harrison, former Assistant Dean of Boston University's School of Medicine and Chief Medical Officer at Washington, DC's General Hospital has been in medical practice for over twenty-five years. She has come to be recognized as an astute physician who looks at her patient as an entire person. During her medical training at the University of Maryland, Harvard University, and Boston University, she masterfully grasped the traditional side of medicine. She put this knowledge into practice and has helped many from her expertise.

During the last twelve years, she has widened her field of learning and practice to holistic medicine. Dr. Harrison feels that this has opened up more opportunities to do as the Hippocratic oath states, "do no harm."

Dr. Harrison did not immediately embrace TAHITIAN NONI® Juice upon hearing about it for the first time. In fact, Dr. Harrison has always found, as a medical doctor, there is really not enough time to be able to look into every single new product on the market. In addition, she didn't like pharmaceutical representatives, or others, telling her what to prescribe for her patients. When she strictly practiced conventional methods, pharmaceutical representatives were disappointed when they came into the office to find that she was in charge. They knew her answer to them: "I'll call you if a need arises."

It was the same type of situation when Dr. Harrison began incorporating natural supplements into her medical practice. Approximately every two weeks, Dr. Harrison would get someone wanting her to look at a new herb or natural substance. When Dr. Harrison was introduced to TAHITIAN NONI® Juice, she simply said that she couldn't look at another product at the moment.

However, some members of her staff began using the juice personally, and they started having wonderful results. They urged her to take a closer look at the ancient Polynesian plant called *Morinda citrifolia.* So she did. At first, Dr. Harrison used it with just a few of her patients who were slowly moving back to better health. When these patients responded so well and so quickly to the juice, Dr. Harrison began to think that there was something special about the juice.

Now she uses noni with a number of her patients, particularly those who have a very complicated history. Dr. Harrison has also published a book on noni entitled *What Else Every Doctor Should Know: An Introduction to Noni and the Brains.*[30]

In her book, Dr. Harrison explains that she believes some of the components in noni have a remarkable ability to cross cell membranes and the blood brain barrier. She bases it on the research done by Drs. Michael Frost and Owens Moore.[32,33] One of her main points about noni is that she believes it helps boost the function of the pineal gland, which is a critical part to the overall well-being of the body. The pineal gland is directly in charge of the body's production and distribution of the neurohormones, melatonin, and serotonin. These compounds affect a myriad of functions and organs within the body. If a person's pineal gland is running at optimum, then, in turn, the body should function better.

Dr. Harrison explains, "The pineal gland is responsible for one's biological clock. Substances it secretes allow for a good night's sleep... People may lose weight when these substances are present. Some find that they don't get weakened bones or teeth... They don't get infections and tumors tend to shrink away. Bowel movements are regular...They have plenty of energy. All of these results from a fully functioning pineal gland are the same things I hear in the testimonials of my patients and others who have taken TAHITIAN NONI® Juice." [34]

Robert Fischer, MD

Dr. Robert Fischer, a specialist at The Aesthetic Plastic Surgery Center of New Jersey in Fort Lee, has been in practice since 1972. His specialty is Plastic and Reconstructive Surgery. For the past few years he recommended that patients take bromelain, grape seed extract, and *Arnica montana* to decrease swelling and bruising peri-operatively. However, recently Dr. Fischer has switched to having his patients take TAHITIAN NONI® Juice several weeks before elective surgery, and as soon as possible after emergency procedures.

Dr. Fischer says the results he sees with TAHITIAN NONI® Juice are what he was hoping to see before with the previous regimen. Not only are the benefits from noni dramatically visible, but also he is seeing a markedly reduced need for post-op analgesics. In addition, he is seeing significant reduction in recovery time and convalescence.

Dr. Fischer began using noni in his practice after personally using the juice on a daily basis for two and half years. His elective cosmetic and reconstructive surgical patients are encouraged to drink a loading dose of 2 ounces of noni twice a day for three or four weeks prior to their surgery. Patients then continue using it post-op until fully recovered. Dr. Fischer has been noticing virtually pain-free and faster recoveries from some very major procedures, and he attributes it to the diminished reaction of the tissues to the trauma of surgery. TAHITIAN NONI® Juice helps the patient to incur less bruising and swelling through its natural analgesic and antibiotic properties. Noni also seems to help bolster the immune system, which is never a bad thing before surgery.
Dr. Fischer finds that patients, who would ordinarily require a transfusion or several weeks to get back on their feet, are now recovering without the transfusion in much quicker time.

Dr. Gary Tran

Dr. Gary Tran has been a practicing veterinarian in the United States for nearly twenty-six years. He graduated from Oklahoma State University, College of Veterinary Medicine in 1964. Like many other American-trained veterinarians, he was schooled in using conventional therapeutics. A few years into his practice, he took a trip to his homeland of Vietnam and saw other modalities (acupuncture, herbal medicine) that were being used with documented success. He was amazed at what these alternative methods were doing in third-world countries where drugs are sometimes in short supply and usually very expensive.

After seeing with his own eyes what alternative modalities could do, he knew he wanted to try to incorporate some of them into his American practice. In addition, he learned that these methods seemed to help patients suffering from diseases that usually drugs couldn't touch such as viral infections, organ failure problems, chronic degenerative diseases, and cancers.

Since that time, he has been using integrative veterinary medicine. In 1997, Dr. Tran was introduced to TAHITIAN NONI® Juice. At first he was skeptical of all the seemingly broad-spectrum claims of its therapeutic reach. Upon using it, however, Dr. Tran discovered noni's versatility and therapeutic potency. After five years of using noni in his practice, Dr. Tran has seen first-hand how this supplement is important in helping maintain better health in animals. In addition, he has found the juice to be extremely safe.

He estimates having used the juice on about 9,000 of his patients (animals). He believes TAHITIAN NONI® Juice works best against debilitating chronic inflammatory diseases (degenerative osteoarthritis, hip dysplasia, spinal disk syndrome, lick granuloma). However, he has found it to also be useful with the following conditions with or without conventional therapeutics:

- intractable immune system failure conditions (auto-immune hemolytic anemia, lupus erythematosus, feline asthma, severe skin allergies, antibiotic-resistant chronic infections, Irritable Bowel Disease)

- life-threatening organ failure problems (congestive heart failure, kidney failure, liver failure, necrotizing pancreatitis)

- untreatable severe viral infections (feline leukemia, feline infectious peritonitis, feline AIDS, parvoviral infection, coronaviral infection)

- incurable neoplastic diseases (squamous cell carcinoma, mast cell tumor, melanoma, hemangiosarcoma, prostate cancer)

- neurological diseases (vestibular syndrome, seizure of all types, ischemic stroke, heat stroke, neurological deficit of all type)

- trauma (brain concussion, brain edema, sprain, fractures, shock, internal bleeding, pulmonary contusion)

- toxicoses (snake bite, spider venom, mushroom poisoning, plant poisoning, rat poisoning, massive bee sting, drug toxicoses)

- surgical support (prevention of anesthetic accidents, prevention of post-surgical infections, promotion of rapid and uneventful healing, elimination of post-surgical pain)

Dr. Tran says that while a few veterinarians have not approved of his use of noni, many of his open-minded colleagues actually send their "incurable" patients to him because he usually sends them back "alive and cured."

Dr. Tran urges other veterinarians to research the possibility of adding alternative veterinary medicine modalities to their conventional therapeutic armamentarium against diseases that are intractable to conventional therapeutics. Dr. Tran believes there are nutraceuticals, such as TAHITIAN NONI® Juice, that are safe and effective to help fight a multitude of disease conditions as well as, if not better than, any drug available. Of course, he stresses that there is always a place for drugs in our fight against diseases, especially when life-threatening symptoms have to be suppressed quickly.

Orlando Pile, MD

Dr. Orlando Pile, a practicing internist for 22 years in Inglewood, California, is the Chief of Communicable Diseases for the Los Angeles Sheriff Department-County Jail. He has served in this position for the last fourteen years. Dr. Pile began incorporating healthy measures into his own life about five years ago. At the time, Dr. Pile, a graduate of College of Medicine and Dentistry of New Jersey, Rutgers Medical School, decided to become a vegetarian as well as try a few other methods to hopefully help improve his own health. About this time he heard an advertisement for noni on the radio. He thought it sounded interesting, but decided not to follow up.

He continued hearing about noni via the radio and other sources, so he finally decided to give it a try. In January of 1998, he took his first swallow of Morinda's TAHITIAN NONI® Juice. He was hoping taking the juice would lower his blood pressure or at least give him some "burst" of energy.

Two months went by and Dr. Pile continued to drink the juice daily. Nothing much seemed to happen. Then, one day while driving with his wife, he heard several testimonials from an audiocassette tape about TAHITIAN NONI® Juice. He began telling his wife that he had been drinking the juice with no effects for two months when his wife interrupted him and asked how long it had been since he had had back pain.

Dr. Pile suffered a herniated lumbar disk in an auto accident in 1995. Dr. Pile thought for a minute, and then realized he hadn't had back pain at all ever since he began drinking noni juice. He was so focused on some big miracle to happen that he didn't notice other positive benefits. Shortly after the conversation with his wife, Dr. Pile attended a golf tournament in Las Vegas. He took noni before and after playing golf and he didn't have to take one painkiller. That was the first time in three years he had been able to play golf without taking a pain pill. (As a note, several Olympic medalists also drink TAHITIAN NONI® Juice.)

Dr. Pile decided to start sharing the juice with a few select patients. He quickly started receiving positive feedback from them. Several patients who had hypertension saw a reduction. Type II insulin-dependent diabetics were able to lower their insulin doses, and Type II non-insulin dependent diabetics could either reduce the dose of their medications or even discontinue it.

Some patients with arthritis and lupus erythematosus reported less pain. Patients with anxiety were more relaxed and slept more soundly after drinking the juice regularly. A prostate cancer patient experienced a lowering of his PSA level from 16 to 9.12. Dr. Pile even had a terminally ill AIDS patient who gained 70 pounds after drinking the juice and whose CD4 count increased from 25 to above 200 and whose viral load decreased from 225,000 to 2,000.

Dr. Pile continues to use mostly a western approach to his medical practice. However, he says he has finally realized it is possible, and he believes smart, to incorporate some alternative approaches (like TAHITIAN NONI® Juice) into his work with patients. He believes it creates a well-rounded approach to some of the more difficult medical cases that are becoming much more common.

SECTION IV

Questions
and
Answers

Q. **How does TAHITIAN NONI® Juice help fight cancer?**

A. Dr. Anne Hirazumi Kim's published work shows that noni is an immune system modulator, and it has indirect anti-tumor activity through strengthening cells of the immune system, and allowing them to more efficiently fight cancer. One of the ways it accomplishes it is through increasing macrophage activity, which invade pathogens. Dr. Hirazumi Kim has been studying noni and specifically cancer for more than a decade at the University of Hawaii.

Q. **Would Dr. Hirazumi Kim's work indicate that noni may cause problems for people with autoimmune system diseases, allergies, or organ transplants?**

A. No, as a matter of fact, it should help. According to Dr. Anne Hirazumi Kim's data, noni acts as an immunomodulator, not as an immune system stimulator. Components in noni enhance the positive aspects of the immune system while inhibiting the negative immune responses such as allergic reactions. It also suppresses autoantibodies.[35]

Q. **Are there any published studies to show that TAHITIAN NONI® Juice can protect against carcinogens?**

A. Yes. Dr. Mian-Ying Wang published work shows that TAHITIAN NONI® Juice protects against carcinogens in rats. Her research involves introducing known carcinogens and monitoring the damage to the DNA in the cells of various organs. In male rats, TAHITIAN NONI® Juice provided 60 percent protection in the heart, 50 percent protection in the lungs, 70 percent protection in the liver, and 90 percent in the kidneys. She is now studying human subjects who are heavy smokers. Preliminary data show that TAHITIAN NONI® Juice is a powerful defense against damage to DNA.[36]

Q. **Have any scientists found that TAHITIAN NONI® Juice is a selective COX 2 inhibitor?**

A. Yes, Dr Chen Shu, part of the research team headed by Jarakae Jensen of the Morinda Research Laboratory, under the direction of Stephen Story, showed TAHITIAN NONI® Juice to be a better selective COX 2 inhibitor than most of the N-SAIDS such as aspirin and Ibuprofen. Independent laboratories found that when comparing the percentage Inhibition Ratio of COX 1 to COX 2, TAHITIAN NONI® Juice compared favorably with Vioxx" and Celebrex". TAHITIAN NONI® Juice had literally no side effects. Brett West, a member of the research team, found that TAHITIAN NONI® Juice was valuable in the treatment of arthritis through reduction of inflammation and pain.

Q. **If TAHITIAN NONI® Juice is such a good selective COX 2 inhibitor, can it be used to treat migraine headaches?**

A. Lawrence Jenkyn, MD, Associate Professor of Medicine (Neurology) and Psychiatry at Dartmouth Medical School, presented a lecture at the International Morinda Convention, April 17-21, 2001 in Salt Lake City, UT, where he spoke about the prevalence of lost workdays from migraine headaches. He cited that in the United States, approximately 270 working days per year are lost per 1000 migraine sufferers. He shared some preliminary results and postulated a noni/serotonin relationship. His studies suggest that TAHITIAN NONI® Juice was clinically successful in the treatment of migraines.

Q. Has TAHITIAN NONI® Juice been used to treat addictions?

A. Yes. Dr. William McPhilamy, Ph.D., LN, a Board Certified Addictions Specialist and Licensed Nutritionist, has reported success in using TAHITIAN NONI® Juice to help in the treatment of addiction to heroine, cocaine, marijuana, nicotine, alcohol, prescription drug use, and caffeine.[37]

Q. Has anyone used TAHITIAN NONI® Juice successfully to treat animals?

A. Dr. Gary Tran, DVM, and other veterinarians have had much success. Dr. Tran believes that TAHITIAN NONI® Juice has helped different types of animals with different problems such as bone, joint and muscle conditions, cancer, immune failure, organ failure and most degenerative diseases. Recommended dose schedules for animals and humans can be found in *TAHITIAN NONI® Juice, How Much, How Often, For What.*[38]

Q. How can TAHITIAN NONI® Juice be so successful against such an array of conditions? Is it an antioxidant?

A. Scott Gerson, MD, Clinical Professor at the Mt. Sinai School of Medicine in New York, joins a list of physicians who believe that TAHITIAN NONI® Juice is a powerful antioxidant that also acts as an adaptogen. Gerson believes it is the premiere adaptogen, which has a global balancing effect on all the systems of the human body. He has cited data that show that TAHITIAN NONI® Juice is a more powerful antioxidant than Vitamins C, E, grape seed extract, and Pycnogenol®.

Q. **What do people mean when they talk about noni rejuvenating cellular growth, and its relation to Dr. Heinicke's xeronine system?**

A. Dr. Heinicke believes xeronine is involved in the proper formation of proteins. His proposed xeronine theory explains how noni acts as a cellular protein enhancer. Some scientists believe that xeronine is a critical alkaloid, which the body needs to help repair and create new cells. Dr. Heinicke postulated that proxeronine, under the influence of the enzyme proxeroninease, transforms into xeronine, an alkaloid. Proxeronine is the rate-limiting factor. After more than fifty years of study on the subject, Dr. Heinicke has found that the noni fruit contains the most abundant supply of proxeronine, more than any other known food source. It also contains some already formed xeronine.[39]

Q. **How do you best summarize noni?**

A. It's God's gift to man.

APPENDIX A

Partial Listing of Dr. Solomon's Published Works

Solomon, N., and G. Sayers: "Effect of Temperature and Corticosteroids on Work Capacity of Rat Heart-Lung Preparation." Fifth Interim Scientific Session of the American Rheumatism Association. 1958. *Arthritis and rheumatism*, 1958, 2:376.

Solomon, N., R.H. Travis, and G. Sayers "Corticosteroids and Work Capacity of Rat Heart-Lung Preparation." *Federation Proceedings*, 1958, 17:152.

Solomon, N., and G. Sayers: "Corticosteroids and the Functional Capacity of the Rat Heart Preparation." *Endocrinology*, 1959, 64:535.

Solomon, N., and G. Sayers: "Aldosterone Lanatoside C and Isolated Rat Heart," *Arthritis and Rheumatism*, 1960.

Solomon, N., H.B. Markowitz and G. Sayers: "Corticosteroids and Work Capacity of the Isolated Rat Heart Preparation." First International Congress of Endocrinology, Copenhagen, Denmark, 1960, 825.

Solomon, N., and G. Sayers: "Effects of Corticosteroids on Myocardial Function." Conference on the Human Adrenal Cortex, Glasgow, Scotland, 1960, 32.

Gregerman, R.I., and N. Solomon: "Acceleration of Thyroxine Turnover During Febrile Illness: Evidence for Increased Thyroidal Thyroxine Secretion." *Clinical Research*, April 1964.

Lichtalen, P.R., N. Solomon, L. Bernstein, G.C. Friesinger, and R.S. Ross: "Inotropic Effect of Aldosterone on the Myocardium of Normal Dogs." *Federal Proceedings*, April 1964.

Solomon, N., R.I. Gregerman, and N.W. Shock: "Aging and the Functional Capacity of the Rat Heart-Lung Preparation." *The Gerontologist*, 1964, 4:1E.

C.C.J. Carpenter, N. Solomon, S.G. Silverberg, T. Bledsoe, R.C. Northcutt, J.R. Klinenberg, I.L. Bennett, and A.M. Harvey: "Schmidt's Syndrome (Thyroid and Adrenal Insufficiency) A Review of the Literature and A Report of Fifteen New Cases, Including Ten Instances of Co-existent Diabetes Mellitus." *Medicine*, 1964, 43:153.

Solomon, N., and C.C.J. Carpenter, I.L. Bennett, and A.M. Harvey: " Schmidt's Syndrome (Thyroid and Adrenal Insufficiency) and the Co-existence of Diabetes Mellitus." *Diabetes*, 1965, 14:300.

Solomon, N., P.S. Aughenbaugh, R.I. Gregerman, and N.W. Shock: "Aging and the Functional Capacity of the Rat Heart-Lung Preparation." *The Gerontologist*, 5:39, 1965.

Wagner, H., Jr., T. Migita, and N. Solomon: "Effect of Age on Reticuloendothelium Function in Man." J. Gerontology, 1966, 21, No. 1:57.

Solomon, N.: *The Bulletin of the Maryland Dietetic Association,* "Weight Loss Through Food Withdrawal." Vol. 18, No. 2:3, 1966.

Gregerman, R.I. and N. Solomon: "Acceleration of Thyroxine and Triiodothyronine Turnover During Bacterial Pulmonary Infections and Fever: Implications for the Functional State of the Thyroid During Stress and In Senescence." *Journal of Clinical Endocrinology and Metabolism,* January 1967, 27: (1) 91-1 n4.

Solomon, N., N.W. Shock, A. Davidoff, S. Winkler, and M.H.M. Lee, (Eds.) *Dentistry for the Special Patient: The Aged, Chronically Ill, and handicapped* – Chapter 2, Physiology of Aging, Philadelphia – London – Toronto: W.B. Saunders Co. 1966.

Solomon, N.: "Studying and Treating the Obese Patient." *Maryland State Medical Journal,* May 1968, 17:64-69.

Solomon, N.: "The Study and Treatment of the Obese Patient." *Hospital Practice,* March 1969, 4:90-94.

Solomon, N., and N.W. Shock: "Nutrition in the Aged." *Southern Medical Journal,* December 1969, 62, No. 12:1523-28.

Solomon, N.: "A Message from the Secretary of Health and Mental Hygiene," *Maryland's Health,* March 1979, 42, No. 1:2.3.

Solomon, N., and N.W. Shock: "Nutrition in the Aged." *Southern Medical Journal,* March 1970, 63, No. 3:274-79.
Solomon, N., N.W. Shock, and Patricia S Aughenbaugh: "The Daily Needs and Interest of Older People," *The Biology of Aging,* 1970. Fort Lauderdale, Florida, Charles C. Thomas, Chapter 10.

Solomon, N., M. Tayback: "State of the State's Health," *Maryland State Medical Journal,* July 1970, 19, No. 7:48-50.

Solomon, N.: "The National Scene," *Maryland State Medical Journal,* August 1970, 19, No. 8:93.

Solomon, N., and Matthew Tayback: "Family Health Assurance," *American Journal of Public Health,* September 1970, 60, No. 9:1678-80.
Solomon, N.: "The Communication Gap and the Drug Problem," *Maryland State Medical Journal.* November 1970, 19, No. 11:78-81.

Solomon, N., and Matthew Tayback: "Care of the Aged," *Maryland State Medical Journal,* November 1970, 19, No. 11105-06.

Solomon, N., and Matthew Tayback: "New Programs for the Mentally Retarded," *Maryland State Medical Journal*, November 1970 19. No. 11-108.

Solomon, N., and Matthew Tayback: "The Care of the Mentally Subnormal," *Maryland State Medical Journal*, January 1971, 20, No. 1:79.

Solomon, N.: "Home Health Services in the Care of the Chronically Ill," *Maryland State Medical Journal*, January 1971, 20, No. 1: 79.

Solomon, N.: "Major Legislative Proposals," *Maryland State Medical Journal*, March 1971, 20, No. 3:83.

Solomon, N., and George J. Dendrinos: "Current Diagnosis –Section 9," Disorders of Metabolism – Obesity, 1971, Philadelphia – London – Toronto; W.B. Saunders Co.

Solomon, N.: "Health Hazards of Obesity." *Obesity and Bariatric Medicine*, May-June 1972, 1, No. 1:3-5.

Solomon, N.: "Fad, Crash Diet May Work Temporarily, at a High Risk," *Family Practice News*, May 15, 1973, Volume III, No. 10.

Solomon, N.: "Improper Dieting – Health Hazard," *Maryland State Medical Journal*, April 1974, 23, 4:70.

Solomon, N.: "An Exchange Diet for Your Patients," *Maryland State Medical Journal*, September 1974, 23, 7:47-50.

Solomon, N.: "The Jewish Tradition of Justice," *The Lamp*, April 1975, 22, No. 2.

Solomon, N.: "Swine Flu – The Whole Story," *The Los Angeles Times Syndicate*. Los Angeles, October 1976.

Solomon, N.: "The Plain Talk About Weight Loss," *The Los Angeles Times Syndicate*, January 1977.

Solomon, N., and Robert Dershewitz: "The Relationship of Weight Loss to Blood Pressure in the Obese, Hypertensive Adolescent," *Maryland State Medical Journal*, June 1981, 30, 60:56-56.

Solomon, N., and W. Tichenor: "The Role of Food Allergies in Obesity," *Maryland State Medical Journal*, October 1980, 100.

Solomon, N., with Gary Nyman: "Mental Hygiene Within the State Health Care Delivery System: The Maryland Perspective," *Maryland State Medical Journal*, 1980, 29, 6:62-66.

Tichenor, W.S., and N. Solomon: "Cessation of Smoking," *Journal of American Medical Association*, January 23/30, 1981, 245: No. 4.

Solomon, N.: *Findings on Needle Park: Switzerland's Social Experiment with Legalizing Drugs.* Report to Governor William Donald Schaefer, Annapolis, Maryland, December 4, 1991.

Solomon, N. and M. Bellmore: Conclusions of the Second Report to the Governor of The Solomon Commission on Health Care Reform in Maryland. Report to Governor William Donald Schaefer, Annapolis, Maryland, Spring, 1993.

Passwater, R. and N. Solomon: *The Case For Preventive Nutrition* Audio tape, Living Better Longer. Edmond, Oklahoma, Health Solutions, 1996.

Passwater, R. and Solomon, N.: *Experts' Optimal Health Journal*, Vol. 1, Issue 5: Homocystine, Risk Factor for Heart Disease and Cancer. Montreal, Canada, Apprise Publications, 1997.

Passwater, R. and Solomon, N.: Experts' Optimal Health Journal, Vol. 1, Issue 6: Iron Overload Disorders: Deadly to Millions of North Americans. Montreal, Canada, Apprise Publications, 1997.

Solomon, N. and Udall, C.: *The Noni Phenomenon.* ISBN 1-887938-87-7. Vineyard, UT: Direct Source Publishing, Inc., 1999.

Solomon, N., R. Passwater, and R Elkins: *Soy Smart Health* Pleasant Grove, UT: Woodland Publishing, 2000.

Solomon, N.: Nobel Prize Winner, Dr. Paul Zane Pilzer, Commentary by Neil Solomon, M.D., Ph.D. *The Next Trillion $ Seceret* Audiotape. Vineyard, UT: Sound Concepts, 2001.

ENDNOTES

1 – Alexandra Dittmar, "Morinda citrifolia L. Use in Indegenous Samoan Medicine," Journal of Herbs, Spices and Medical Plants, Vol. 1(3), 1993.

2 – Ibid.

3 – Solomon, N. and Udall, C. The Noni Phenomenon. ISBN 1-887938-87-7. Vineyard, UT: Direct Source Publishing, Inc., 1999.

4 – Bushnell, O.A., et al. "The Antibacterial Properties of Some Plants Found in Hawaii." Pacific Science 4:167-183 (1950).

5 – F.L. Tabrah and B.M. Eveleth, "Evaluation of the Effectiveness of Ancient Hawaiian Medicine," Hawaii Medical Journal, Vol. 25, 1966.

6 – Agarwal, K. K. "Preliminary Pharmocological Studies with the Extract of Morinda citrifolia." Indian Journal of Physiology & Pharmacology 12:21 (1967).

7 – Levand, O and Larson, H. O. "Some Chemical Constituents of Morinda citrifolia." Planta Medica 36(2): 186-187 (1979).

8 – Abbott, I.A., and C. Shimazu. "The Geographic Origin of the Plants most Commonly Used for Medicine by Hawaiians." Journal of Ethnopharmacology 14 (1985).

9 – Solomon, Neil. The Noni Phenomenon, Direct Source Publishing: Vineyard, Utah, 1999.

10 – E-mail correspondence from Maria Odegbaro, M.D.

11 – ibid.

12 – ibid.

13 – E-mail correspondence with Dr. Richard Dicks.

14 – Personal correspondence with Jarakae Jensen.

15 – Chafique Younos, Alain Rolland, Jacques Fleurentin, Marie-Claire Lanhers, Rene Misslin, and Francois Mortier, "Analgesic and Behvioural Effects of Morinda citrifolia," Planta Med, Vol. 56, 1990.

16 – Hirazumi, Anne. "Antitumor Studies of a Traditional Hawaiian Medicinal Plant, Morinda citrifolia (Noni). In Vitro and In Vivo." Doctoral dissertation, Universtiy of Hawaii: 1997.

17 – Phytother Res 1999 Aug; 12(5): 380-7.

18 – A. Hirazumi, E. Furusawa, S.C. Choud, and Y. Hokama, "Anti-cancer Activity of Morinda citrifolia (Noni) on Intraperitoneally Implanted Lewis Lung Carcinoma in Syngeneic Mice," Proc. West Pharmacol. Soc. Vol. 376, 1994.

19 – Tomonori Hiramatsu, Masaya Imoto, Takashi Koyano, Kazuo Umezawa, "Induction of Normal Phenotypes in Ras-Transformed Cells by Damnacanthal from Morinda citrifolia," Cancer Letters, Vol. 73, 1993.

20 – Y. Asahina et al. "Effect of Okadaic acid and noni fruit extract in the synthesis of tumor necrosis factor alpha by peripheral blood mononuclear." Proceedings of the International Symposium of Ciguatera and Marine Natural Products: 197-205.

21 – M.Y. Wang, W. Bender, and L.F. Yu. "Preventive Effects of Tahitian Noni Juice on the Formation of 7, 12-demethylbenz(a)anthracene (DMBA) DNA Adducts in vivo." Submitted to The American Association for Clinical Research, AACR 91st Annual Meeting: April 1-4, 2000, San Francisco.

22 – Wang, M.Y. and C. Su. "Cancer Prevention: Molecular Mechanisms to Clinical Applications," Vol. 952, 161-168. Annals of the New York Academy of Sciences, Dec. 2001.

23 – E-mail correspondence from Dr. Kenneth Stejskal.

24 – E-mail correspondence from Joel Fuhrman.

25 – "Noni Plant May Yield New Drugs To Fight Tuberculosis," HONOLULU, Dec. 18, 2000. (Report of the findings at the 2000 International Chemical Congress of Pacific Basin Societies held in Honolulu, Hawaii.)

26 –   Solomon, Neil. The Noni Phenomenon, Direct Source Publishing: Vineyard, Utah, 1999.

27 –   Heinicke, Ralph. The Xeronine System: A New Cellular Mechanism that Explains the Health Promoting Action of Noni and Bromelain. Direct Source Publishing: Orem, Utah, 2001.

28 –   1998 Nobel Prize winners: Drs. Robert Fuchgott, Ferid Murad, and Louis Ignarro, Stockholm, Sweden.

29 –   1999 Nobel Prize winner: Gunther Blobel, Stockholm, Sweden.

30 –   Hall, Steven. Noni Through Your Body. Orem, Utah: Direct Source Publishing, 1999.

31 –   Harrison, Mona. What Else Every Doctor Should Know: An Introduction to Noni and the Brains. Orem, Utah: Direct Source Publishing, 2002.

32 –   Moore, T. Owens, Ph.D., The Science of Melanin Dispelling the Myth, Silver Springs, MD; Ventura Books/ Beckland House Publishers, Inc., 1995.

33 –   Frost, Michael. Ph.D. Choosing Life Ways, Press, Richmond Heights, OH, 1947.

34 –   Harrison, Mona. What Else Every Doctor Should Know: An Introduction to Noni and the Brains. Orem, Utah: Direct Source Publishing, 2002.

35 –   Phytother Res 1999 Aug; 12(5): 380-7.

36 –   Wang, M.Y. and C. Su. "Cancer Prevention: Molecular Mechanisms to Clinical Applications," Vol. 952, 161-168. Annals of the New York Academy of Sciences, Dec. 2001.

37 –   McPhilamy, William. Noni and Addictions: A Way Out, Direct Source Publishing: Orem, Utah, 2001.

38 –   Solomon, Neil. TAHITIAN NONI® Juice, How Much, How Often, For What, Direct Source Publishing: Orem, Utah, 2000.

39 –   Heinicke, Ralph. The Xeronine System: A New Cellular Mechanism that Explains the Health Promoting Action of Noni and Bromelain. Direct Source